Pamela Williams

Living with Migraines

Understanding Migraines and Your Triggers, While Staying Positive and Living Life to the Fullest

This book was professionally typeset on Reedsy
Find out more at *reedsy.com*

I would like to dedicate this book to my parents, David and Barbara Williams

They instilled in me the values and character traits that made me the woman I am today. Dad, thank you for showing me that everything does happen for a reason. I pass that wisdom on to others every chance I get. I miss you Dad! And Mom, thank you for the countless hours you spent with me at Urgent Care for all of my migraines. I love you!

Proverbs 17:22

"A cheerful heart is good medicine, but a crushed spirit dries up the bones"

-The Bible (NIV)

Contents

    1.

    2.

    3.

    4.

    5.

    6.

Introduction

I will start off by saying that I am not a doctor, but I have been a migraine sufferer for almost 35 years, so I feel that makes me somewhat an expert in dealing and living with migraines, in my mind at least. I have been searching for remedies and ways to cope since 1990, and I've definitely realized what works for one person will not for the next. I have always been proactive with my Neurologist and I ask a lot of questions. I also do a lot of research online to get tips and ideas to see what can help me. With that being said, I've seen so many books about migraines. I thought to myself; what is a better way to feel empowerment and take charge of my life than by writing my own migraine book? So here I am.

It comes down to understanding migraines and what they really are. Do you know exactly what kind of migraines you get? Or do you want to understand them for a loved one? Understanding migraines is the first step in taking control in your life. It's the dice I rolled, so I better make the best of it.

The next step is finding a doctor or Neurologist that you are comfortable with. When you have your migraines diagnosed, you should be starting pain management care with your doctor. There are so many medications that can treat migraines, so it's impossible to discuss all of them. Your doctor and books by doctors can get into details about what all there is to offer. Bottom line, if you choose medication as part of your pain management journey, it comes down to trial and error with those medications. This book is not about what you should be taking, but rather a quick guide or a checklist of battling this monster so you control it rather than it controlling you. I don't know about you, but when I meet people, I want to be known as "Pam", not Pam who has migraines". I would be ok with "Pam the ninja" or the "tattooed chick", but that's for another book in the making perhaps lol.

With your health care, it is not just up to the doctor for your journey. You are responsible for knowing what your triggers are, and for recognizing common symptoms. Many migraine sufferers keep a "migraine journal" to keep track of their migraines and what started it. You learn what affects you and then you can start dealing with it.

Pain management is such a broad term, as there are so many approaches for this. Working with your doctor is a priority and keeping them in the loop of your journey goes a long way in your coping with this monster. Can we call migraines monsters? I think so.

So what are some remedies you can do on your own, without relying on prescription medications? For starters, think about the basics. I'm not talking about the silly "cures" that your friends and loved ones send you, like, "Hey, I saw this online about putting your feet in water to cure your migraine". I'm talking about ice/or heat on your head or neck. There are plenty of herbal remedies and supplements to explore. Everyone talks about the holistic approach. I think there's something to be said for that. There are also many devices and gadgets that can help.

Even with understanding migraines and being on a pain management regimen, there is so much more. It's called support. I know too many people that don't understand. They ask you, "Oh, do you have another headache?" If I had a nickel for every time I heard headache instead of migraine, I'd be rich! I only wish it was just a headache! Find support groups. I never wish ill will on anyone, but there is comfort in knowing that others are going through the same thing as you. I think knowledge and acceptance is the key to taking control of your life.

I know there are so many migraine books out there already, and great books too. Am I saying anything new here in my book? Probably not, but I think we need reminders from time to time that we are not alone. If I was ever going to write a book, I was asked to write down 10 of my favorite things to do. I looked at that list, and of course migraines were not on there. I thought, how can I do everything on my list if I don't take control of my migraines? I will always have them probably, but I remembered, I'm feisty. I got this! Maybe writing this book is just for me to look at this monster dead in the face. But as my dad always used to say, "everything happens for a reason". I have never felt more empowered than before. I can only hope that I haven't suffered all these years for nothing. Maybe someone   can   learn   from   my   journey   thus   far.

1

Understanding Migraines

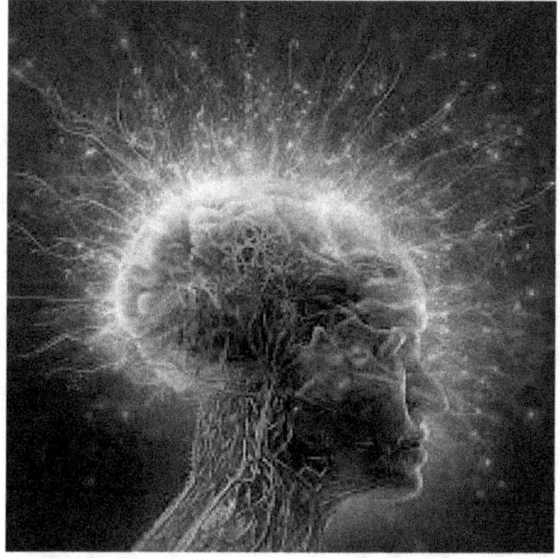

I think the number one question people always ask is, "what is the difference between a headache and a migraine?" A migraine is a headache from hell. Many of my friends don't actually know what a true migraine is. Some do, and they even know when one is coming on even before I do sometimes. I'm sure you've all been there. Friends and family mean well. Some look right at you and tell you to just take Tylenol. I usually just grin and say "thanks".

Here is my meaning in the easiest form I can think of for a migraine. A migraine is an intense headache, but adding on other symptoms to intensify the entire experience. There are many descriptions and diagrams of the difference between a headache and a migraine. I know with my migraines the pain is throbbing and always on one side of my head or the other, and sometimes bounce from the front to back. Now add nausea, and sensitivity to light, sound, and smells. It's very easy to throw up. I sometimes get visual disturbances, which are migraines with aura. The first time I had one, I thought I was having a stroke. I get a flickering light and wavy or zigzag lines that I see that last about 20-30 minutes.

The four stages for a migraine

I've learned that there are four stages for a migraine:

- Prodrome
- Aura
- Attack
- Postdrome

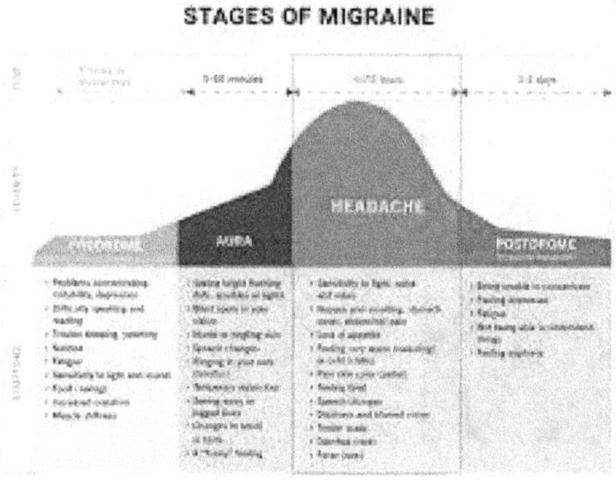

This is basically your before, during and after stages. It took my years to realize that this was actually a thing. It was like a light bulb went off in my head! Ever wonder why you crave certain foods every now and then? Or yawn a lot when you're not tired? How about why you have to pee more than normal? This is the prodrome stage.

I mentioned the visual disturbances I experience. This is the aura stage. This stage happens with maybe 25% of sufferers if I had to guess.

Now the attack stage is what most sufferers already completely understand. This is what a lot of non sufferers think we only experience. This is the pain and side effects, like nausea, and sensitivity to light, sound and smells. This can last from a day to several days.

Once the migraine finally goes away, you are left with the postdrome stage. This is the stage where a lot of people say they have a migraine hangover. You feel like you've been hit by a Mack truck or just ran a marathon. You are wiped out. I know a lot of people experience the prodrome stage symptoms as well during this stage.

I find this to be an ongoing cycle. I deal with a migraine. Get through it. Wait for the next one. It's almost like living on eggshells, but I refuse to let this disease control me. You learn to have a "security blanket" of remedies readily available so you're not caught off guard. I'll get into that more in the pain management chapter.

I almost forgot to mention migraine brain fog. How ironic, huh? This happens during the four stages of a migraine. It can start 48 hours before you get the attack and can easily last 24 after the migraine is over. I have just simply accepted this part about migraines. I used to feel stupid when I couldn't think of words and couldn't focus. I know I can't control this. My brain fog starts in the first stage usually before I get my migraine. Lucky me. My friends usually point out that I'm about to get a migraine. And of course I'm an overachiever, so the fog remains until Postdrome is over. Brain fog is also a side effect of some of the migraine meds. Just keep that in mind.

There are many types of migraines, like one isn't enough, right? By knowing what they are, it might help you or a loved one with the migraine journey.

Types of migraines

Types of migraines:

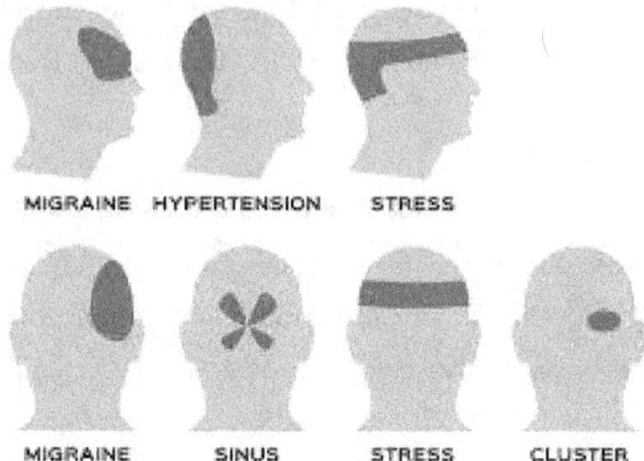

-
- Common and chronic migraines
- A common migraine is when you get an attack a couple times a month maybe. A chronic migraine on the other hand is when you get 15 or more attacks a month. Your day to day life can be greatly impacted.
- Cluster Headache
- More severe than a common migraine but it doesn't last as long, maybe up to a couple hours (more men are prone to this).
- Rebound migraine
- This is when you take medication for too long. This goes for prescription and over-the-counter medications as well. Sometimes the rebound migraine can feel worse than the original migraine itself.
- I find that the only way to get rid of these is one of two ways. You can either go to Urgent Care / ER for meds (this resets me to a zero usually) or you can flush your system of ALL meds. This means over-the-counter meds (OTC) as well. Yes, this takes longer (usually about 5 days), but then your meds work like the first time again.
- Migraine with Aura (Classic Migraine)

- This is when you get the crazy light show to mess with your vision. You see wavy or zigzag lines. This normally does not come with any pain. This comes on suddenly with little to no warning, and lasts usually 20-30 minutes. Sometimes a regular migraine follows.

- Other

(I won't go into details as these are more rare, except menstrual lol, but they are here for you to explore if you think you fall into this category).

- Silent Migraine (Acephalgic)
- Hemiplegic Migraine
- Retinal Migraine
- Menstrual Migraine
- Abdominal Migraine

2

Health Care

Finding the right doctor

First and foremost about living with migraines is making sure you are diagnosed properly and getting medical care for it. You can get as many opinions and suggestions from friends or off the internet, but advocating for your own health is paramount. There are so many variables to migraines, that I really believe you need a doctor or Neurologist in your corner. And don't just sit back and let them do and say everything. This is your head we're talking about! What I mean by that, is asking questions. Why am I taking this medication over that? Do your own research on new medications or treatments and ask about possibilities. You and your doctor need to act as a team to find what works for you.

To date, there is no cure for migraines. No magic wand to make it all better. The easiest way to deal with migraines is medication. I hate taking meds. I keep thinking, "just fix me already!". I've accepted my migraine disease as any other. I say that, but I'm kicking and screaming inside like a kid that didn't get their own way. People with high blood pressure or heart conditions take medications. Same for diabetes and so on.

Abortive and preventative medications

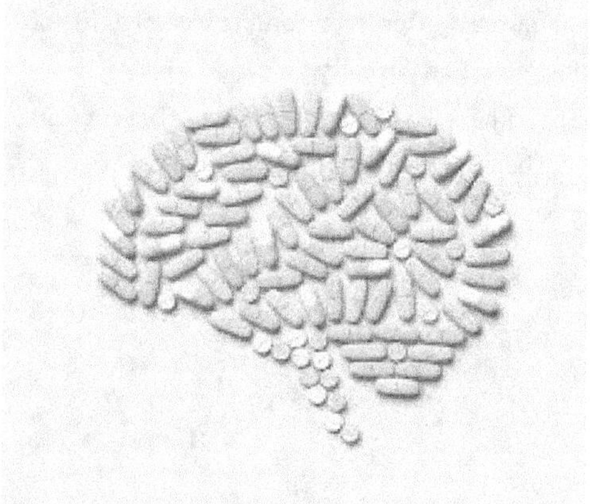

So what are migraine medication options? You can get abortive and preventative medications from your doctor, or you can get over-the-counter (OTC):

- Preventative
- Daily medication to help reduce the frequency and severity of the migraine attack
- Pills, nasal sprays, Botox, etc.
- Abortive (also called Acute or Rescue)
- Medicine to take immediately when the attack comes on. It's usually best to take meds at the onset of the attack. This is why I usually have my "security blanket" of meds with me at all times.
- Over-the-counter
- Many try to deal with their migraines by taking OTC, as it can be cheaper and/or less trips to the doctor for refill prescriptions.

- Urgent Care or ER
- This is always a difficult area to discuss, as everyone gets different care depending on where they go. Most Urgent Cares and hospitals do not like or can't administer strong medication to help you. Unfortunately with today's society, you are dealing with competing with drug addicts coming in just looking for their next fix. So a lot of times you are

treated like a drug seeker when coming in. Many sufferers won't come for that reason, and stay home and suffer. I am fortunate enough to not experience this for the most part. I can usually go in and I get my "cocktail" that works for me. I have Kaiser so I go to their Urgent Care, so they can see my charts. Thankfully I rarely have to go there anymore.

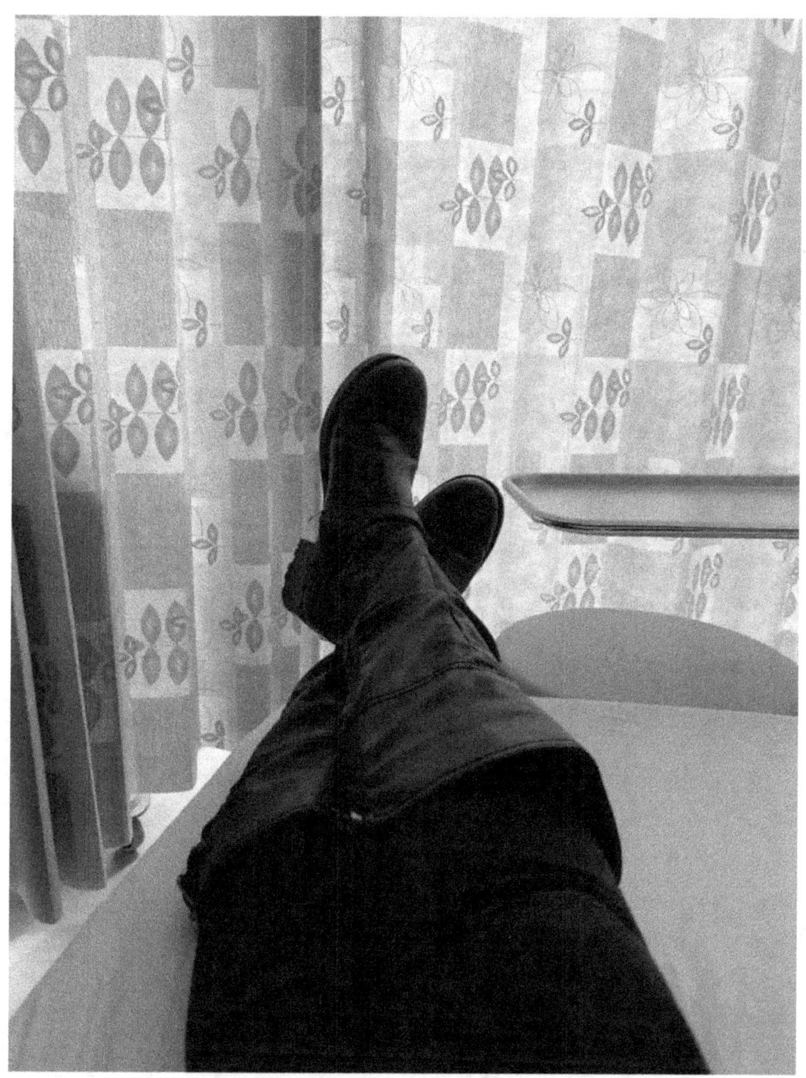

I decided not to go into specific medications here, as this should be between you and your doctor. There's also too many to list. Just know that no matter what kind of medication you choose, there are always pros and cons. And everyone is different. What works for me might not work for someone else. You will find there is trial and error when it comes to medication. It can be as simple as the dosage of a medication to a combination to see what works. I always put it into this perspective; one man's trash is another man's treasure.

I also want to remind people of rebound migraines when taking medications too often. I know so many people on this migraine journey where we are all in the same boat of regulating our meds. You take meds to feel better, but because you had to take them for so many days, now you almost feel worse. I feel like I'm juggling my meds all the time. You know the saying, it's a blessing and curse? Bingo! Welcome to our world.

I can say this for others as well, but having meds is a numbers game every month. Take my Maxalt for instance. I get 12 pills a month. I get about 15 migraines a month. The math doesn't add up, yet I'm forced to make it work. Don't even get me started with my Firoicet. I get a 12 day supply each month. I can take a pill every 6 hours as needed. Of course I have to worry about rebound migraines if I take too much, but I still juggle and ration this medication every month to make sure I last the entire month. Do I really need this today? Does anyone else reason with themselves when deciding what to do? Thankfully I have several abortive meds to choose from, but I am still usually back to square one each month with my supply. There are good days and bad. Good months and bad.

Triggers and common symptoms

This is why understanding your triggers helps a lot. I'm trying to work on my lifestyle to help manage and cope with my migraines. Some triggers you can't escape from, but if I can minimize what I can, I think I'm in a much better place to manage the migraines that I do get. For example, my hormone migraines used to be brutal, but thankfully my gynecologist and neurologist worked together and recommended a full hysterectomy. I have eliminated those types of migraines completely! Now I know everyone can't do this or wouldn't choose this option, but I wanted to give you an example. Another example is teeth grinding. I have a night guard now. I also change up my pillows often, as I wake up with neck strain which triggers the migraine. Fun times.

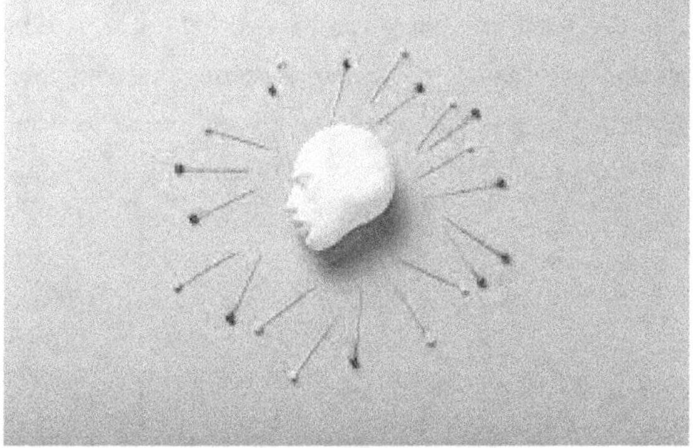

Here are some of the migraine triggers:

- Stress
- Sleep
- Hormones
- Weather
- Diet
- Exercise
- Caffeine & Alcohol
- Dehydration
- Light
- Sound
- Smell
- Teeth Grinding
- Head Injury

- Medication Overuse

The best way to figure out your triggers is to start a migraine journal. You can make your own the old fashioned way and write it down on a log. The easiest way is to get a migraine journal book or download an app. It comes down to preference. In the 90's, I kept a log in a notebook. I tried a migraine app maybe 10 years ago, and it was extremely detailed. While it was a great app, it was very short lived for me, as it was a lot of work in my opinion keeping track of everything. I also basically already knew my triggers, so I was more or less just playing around with the app. But I will say, these can be very helpful if you do not know what your triggers are, and if you are planning on sharing this with your doctor. And let's not forget migraine journal books. The current ones I've seen today look great. I wish these were around when I was first diagnosed!

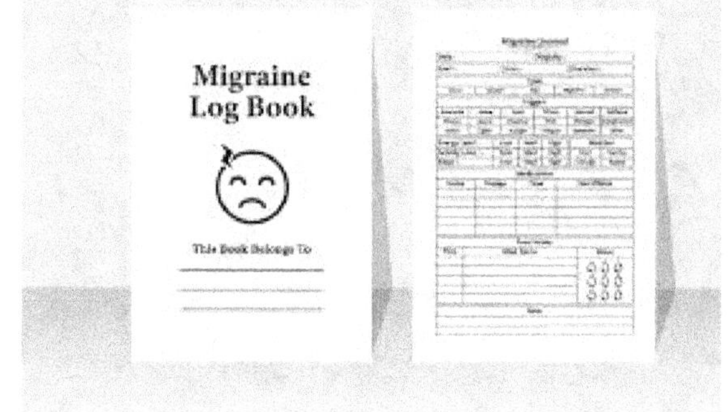

3

Pain Management

When you are at this point in your migraine journey where you have a pain management plan with your doctor and know your triggers, it's almost a fun challenge now for yourself to find your own methods for managing pain to accompany the care plan you have with your doctor. I know what you're thinking right now. Why am I using the word fun and migraines in the same sentence? Well, if you know a thing or two about me, I'm genuinely optimistic. I'm also a realist. I suffer from chronic migraines. I have to take meds. Some days are better than others. But I still put my big boy pants on and live my life every single day to the fullest. So if I can find some other ways to improve my pain without taking meds, I find that amazing. And just like medications being a trial and error, so are finding alternative methods that work for you. So is fun the word to use? Maybe not, but I'm certainly not going to remain negative when I'm searching for things to improve my quality of life. And this means my attitude as well.

When migraines come on, sometimes the simplest of things can help. And once you've been a sufferer for a long time, you almost know in advance if it's going to be a doozy of a migraine, or if you caught it early enough to try a more natural approach before you grab the meds.

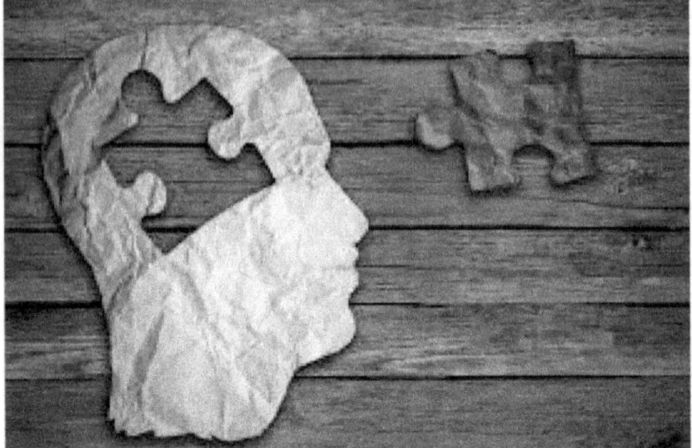

Here's the breakdown of what I think pain management can include:

- **The basics**
- Ice or heat for your head/neck
- Did you drink enough water?
- Add electrolyte powder to your water. This can help with dehydration, and maybe get you to drink more water in general
- Are you getting enough sleep? I keep track of my sleep, so I can gauge the next morning what my day might look like. I also use a sound machine to help me fall asleep and stay asleep.

- **Herbal remedies and supplements**
- If you decide to add some of these to your daily routine, I recommend that you discuss it with your doctor. This way they know what you are taking and that it won't mix with your medication.
- There are also many supplements. I've learned that it was better for me to research on my own what might work. And I've tried many different things over the years. I've changed them up over those years as well. Supplements will also have side effects, so look at the pros and cons of each prior to taking.
- Sinol Nasal Spray - Fast Headache Relief (I found this gem on Amazon recommended by someone in a FB Migraine support group. It's all natural and not habit forming, so a great alternative before grabbing your meds. It's a temporary fix, for a couple hours maybe, but you can

use it multiple times a day. It doesn't work for everyone but it's worth a shot to try. It does have capsaicin in it, so be warned it feels like spraying pepper spray up your nose. This is how I explain it to people: spray, intense pain for literally only 15 seconds if that, your brain is screaming, "what the f*@# did you just do to me?!", and then you suddenly realize your pain went from an 8 to a 3 right after. At least this is my experience every time I take it). Good luck lol!

- **Holistic Approach**
- Essential Oils (find what works for you and smells you can tolerate)
- Avoiding certain foods and alcohol
- Acupressure / Acupuncture
- Herbs and supplements
- Stress management
- Breathing techniques
- Music
- Meditation
- Yoga
- Massage
- Hydration
- Sleep
- Biofeedback and cognitive behavioral therapy

- **Devices and Gadgets**
- Migraine glasses (helps with light sensitivity)
- Therapeutic eye masks (Goggles that can massage around your eyes, and provide heat. Some have music, so check for ones that you can turn music off, as you can be very sensitive to sounds during an attack)
- Acupressure devices
- Grounding mats/sheets
- Cefaly device (external trigeminal nerve stimulation)
- gammaCore (non-invasive vagus nerve stimulation, in the UK, need a prescription)

- sTMS (single pulse transcranial magnetic stimulation, need prescription)
- Embr Wave thermal wristband
- Migraine earplugs (helps with barometric pressure)
- HidrateSpark water bottle

When I know I've tried the basics and it isn't working, I head towards the holistic approach or devices. Have I tried everything on this list? Of course not, but I have tried a lot. With the holistic list, my go-to's are the essential oils, limiting my alcohol, taking some supplements, music, yoga, hydration, and sleep. And this list is just not when I have an attack. I try to live better, and I believe all of these things contribute to less stress in my life.

As far as the devices and gadgets go, I'm always on the lookout for something that might help me. My goal is to be pain free, but the next best thing is not taking as many medications, or having to go to Urgent Care or the ER.

I've talked to many people, and I know they have their favorites with what works for them. I'm sure there are even more things out there on the market than I listed. I've tried a couple different therapeutic eye masks. The first one I got, I was unable to turn the music off. That sound of course intensified my migraine. I then found one that you can turn the music off. I'm able to adjust the massage feeling to pulse or kneading vibrations around the eyes. I can add heat which helps. I found it to be a very relaxing feeling. The sound itself of the mask during the massage reminded me of being in an MRI. I usually add a heating pad on my neck and it's the perfect combination for me.

I kept reading about the Grounding sheets and mat, so I've tried it. It says it's supposed to help. Does it? No clue. But it didn't make it worse. I'll keep trying it. Can't hurt, right?

I have the Cefaly device. It's like a tens unit for your forehead. I call it my Wonder Woman machine because it looks like her tiara. It was a little expensive, but it was one of the best purchases I've made! I've talked to others and it's hit or miss if it works for them. As for me, it helps as a preventative and an abortive.

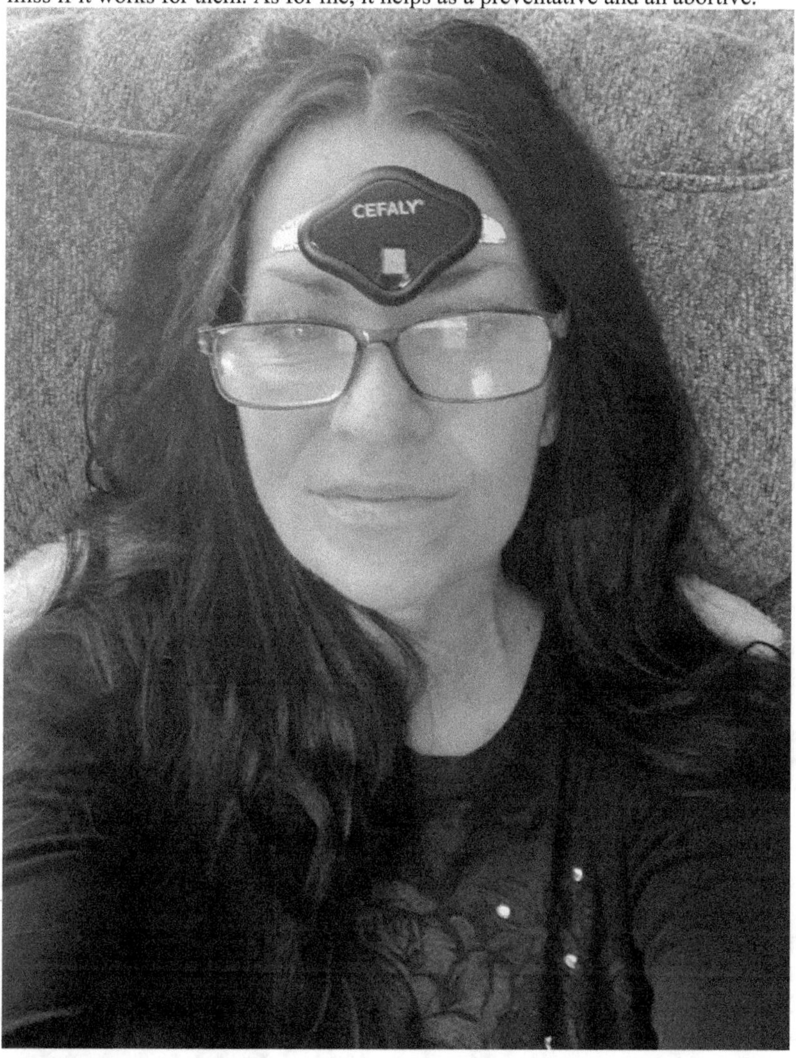

I also have the Embr Wave thermal bracelet. It's like my own little thermometer on my wrist. I can make it warm or cold. This was also a little expensive, but worth every penny to me. For starters, I'm in menopause, so I can make it cold if I'm having a hot flash. However, the main reason I got this is because I am affected by air conditioning pretty badly. I get cold, tense up, get neck strain, and BAM, the migraine comes on. The bracelet acts like holding a hot cup of coffee when you're chilled. It won't warm your core, but it will warm the wrist and I start feeling comfortable.

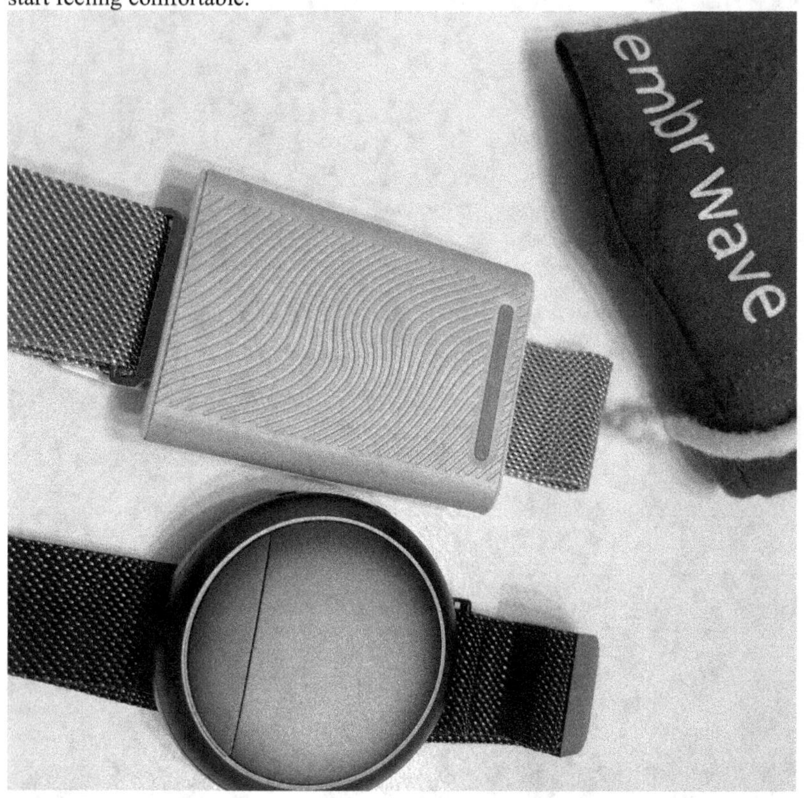

I also have migraine earplugs. These help with the barometric pressure. There's also an app you can download to help track the barometric pressure, and it lets you know when you should put the earplugs in. I have the WeatherX earplugs, but you can also get airplane earplugs which do exactly the same thing. With either earplugs, you can still hear. It just helps with the pressure. I usually wear only one earplug, unless I have a full blown migraine. I still would recommend downloading their app regardless of what earplugs you use, or even if you don't wear the earplugs. There are many times I feel a migraine coming on, and I can't figure out why. I've been good. The weather seems fine. I checked that app and I realized the barometric pressure has changed. The app lets you know ahead of time when the barometric pressure is going to change, so you have a warning.

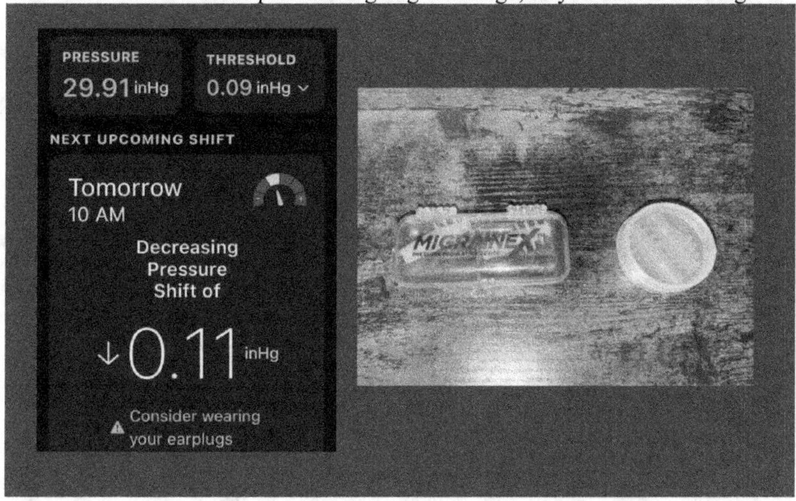

I think many migraine sufferers are in the same boat when trying to cope. You have your health care regimen with your doctor. It constantly needs to be tweaked from time to time. You do your best managing the medications. You figure out your triggers to try to limit the migraines. You add your own pain management to complement the doctor's. All this, mind you, while you may be busy working and running a household, and simply just trying to live your life like everyone else.

4

Finding Support

Some people don't understand you

Even doing everything you're supposed to be doing for your migraines, it sometimes feels hopeless if you don't have support from others. It's easy to feel alone, especially when those around you don't understand. You cancel the plans once again. You can't play with your kids as much as you want. You're living this yet others seem to get annoyed with you. Trust me, I get it. I do what I can when I can. I think the hardest thing about migraine disease is that for the most part, we "look fine" so some people can't grasp when we are completely debilitated from an attack.

And while I'm on the subject of looking fine, there isn't one "look" we have for all of our migraines. There are many times people don't even know we're hurting. Then we can look like we got hit by a Mack truck. I went through some of my pictures over the years to see "my look". I also went back through my Urgent Care visits to see if any correlated. I wonder if you can tell which ones are which. Did I go to Urgent Care for shots? Did I have the migraines for a day? A week? Did I have to call out from work?

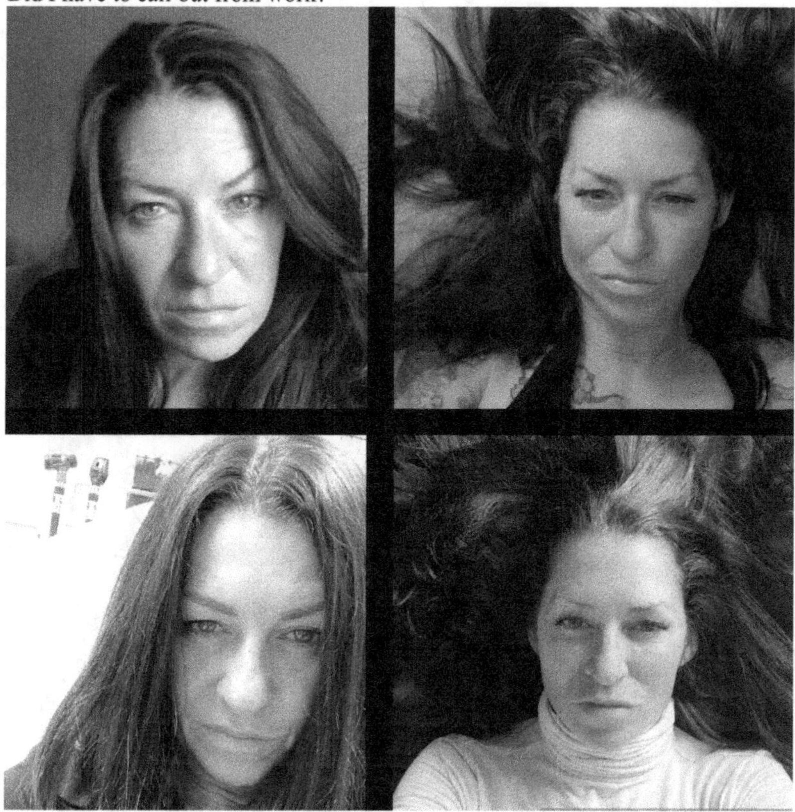

The top left picture:

- I had been fighting that migraine for a week. I was most likely dealing with a rebound migraine at that point. I remember this went on for almost two weeks. I remember a really bad storm came through during this episode also, so barometric pressure was a factor as well. I never went to Urgent Care for this one. Pain was 6-9 the entire time.

The bottom left picture:

- I was working and had to leave work to go to Urgent Care for shots. So since I started work, I must have felt fine and then I got the migraine attack the same day. Pain was 9.

The top right picture:

- This was just my normal migraine. I believe this went on for a day or two. By looking at other pics during that time, I still went to work and still did my normal stuff. I got rid of it with my abortive. Pain was 4-6.

The bottom right picture:

- This was a full blown migraine and I had to go into Urgent Care for shots. Pain was 9.

I don't take a pic every time I have a migraine, as that would be too many pics of me looking crazy. Someone recommended doing it. It might help if you need to show the doctor, in case there are any major changes with the migraines, or drooping of the face or whatever. It kind of made sense so I do it at least a third of the time.

Support groups

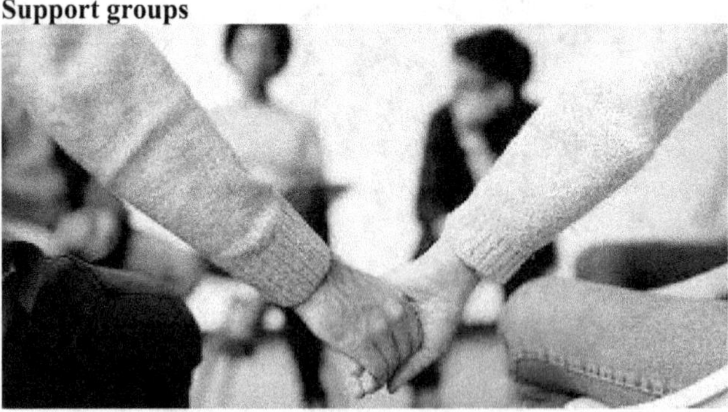

I found Facebook support groups that can really help. They have public and private groups. I know that things I put on the support group page, I do not put on my own page. There's a place for everything. You can get a lot of information from other migraine sufferers, and find out how they are coping. You have to take it with a grain of salt, as everyone has their own opinions of what works. If you are intrigued, then try it. That's what I do. That's how I've learned about new medications and then asked my neurologist to see if I would be a good candidate or not for it. I always try to caution others about praising or bashing a medication because it didn't work for them. It might be a lifesaver for someone else! People often bash a preventative med I take, and it's really helped me. They claim it's the reason they have brain fog. Could be, but as discussed earlier, brain fog comes with the territory of having migraines. You can find out what supplements others are taking. And gadgets; I love gadgets! I've found a few things that work for me all because of a support group.

And then there is simply just searching online for things. The internet is amazing. Type it or voice it, and voila, you get answers to your questions. This is my strategy when I am in a support group. I get a suggestion or recommendation, let's say essential oils that work. They might list two that work for them (lavender and peppermint). I will take it a step further and do my own research about essential oils and see what else might help. There are quite a lot of benefits for migraines with the essential oils. They can help with nausea, sleep, pain, stress, relaxation, and more. I use many different ones depending on my pain level and mood. Also, smell is obviously involved with this so make sure you're ok with it. I know many are very sensitive to smells.

When you think of support, what is a better approach than to start with yourself? I think self-care has been a main focus already in dealing with our physical pain. It's easy to take it a step further with mental and emotional help, as migraines definitely take a toll on the body and mind. I try to focus on the bright side of things. I also use humor to get through tough times. I always have. Yes, I'm one of those types that have a dark sense of humor. I'll also laugh at my friends when they fall down. I will make sure they're ok first (usually). Bottom line, the cards have been dealt. So deal with it. Complaining about it and sulking around will not solve anything. That's my philosophy. I have missed plenty of events due to my migraines. It happens. There have been days where I don't get off the bed or couch. It happens. But I always dust myself off and keep trucking.

The days I can, I go for hobbies and activities of whatever I'm in the mood for. I think it's important to keep your mind busy. There is so much to be said for mindfulness and meditation. And when it's overwhelming at times, reach out for help. It's OK to not be OK. Whether it's a friend, family member, peer support, counseling, you name it.

Advocacy and knowing your rights

One last thing that I'd like to talk about is being an advocate for yourself when it comes to your health. I always thought I was pretty good at that with my doctor. It has, however, taken me a long time to set boundaries socially and at work. You have to know your limits. I have burned the candle at both ends many times for people and especially for my job. So, this is what I have learned. Your friends and family will understand. You can't control it if they don't, and it's not your responsibility to make them. And as far as the job goes, I learned something valuable recently. The organization will always be the organization. You can't be mad when they make a decision, and your feelings don't matter one bit. I have since retired, but I look back and think of everything I did for the job and for coworkers. The time I lost spending with my family. Putting the job before my health. What did it all get me? Nothing. It doesn't matter what your job is. You're replaceable. Accepting that it is what it is, and to let it go will help with your stress level tremendously.

This brings me to knowing what your rights are. I know many sufferers can't work due to their migraines and other conditions. But there are many that do their best to get by and work. I still don't know how I survived my career of almost 24 years before retiring. I know now that I constantly put others before myself. This brings me to FMLA, the Family and Medical Leave Act. I knew of it, but never really understood it until just before I retired. I learned I could have been eligible for this the entire time. I was able to take advantage of it in the last couple months before I left. Looking back, if I had known about this sooner, I think my entire working experience would have been much different and I would have retired much happier. Anyways, I wanted to make sure people were aware of this labor law.

5

Conclusion

I hope you were able to get something out of this book. For a lot of migraine sufferers, this is like an old hat and probably just repetitive. But I'm sure I got some nods along the way of similar experiences or strategies. Maybe I went over something new for you. I will admit that I did have a pretty bad migraine while writing part of this. I didn't let it stop me. I'm just praying I wasn't in a migraine fog at the time lol. I also pray that you think about trying to remain positive while fighting the monster. There really is a lot to be said for being an advocate for your migraine health and living life everyday to the fullest. I for one found it completely empowering sitting down and writing this book.

Thank you for reading my book. It truly means a lot. And if this resonated with you in any way, I would love to hear from you. I would be forever grateful if you could leave me a review on Amazon. Please take care of yourself!

6

Resources

Resourses

12 essential oils for migraine relief. (2015, May 4). Health Central. Retrieved July 14, 2024, from https://www.scribbr.co.uk/referencing/generator/folders/1wzVmRfBz0qfA8Hejm7XnY/lists/7sr7x7iI7KHl723r8H4bQi/

American Migraine Foundation. (2022a, November 29). *Migraine, brain fog and memory loss: How they affect you.* https://americanmigrainefoundation.org/resource-library/migraine-brain-fog/#:~:text=Brain%20fog%20can%20also%20last,as%20a%20%E2%80%9Cmigraine%20hangover.%E2%80%9D

American Migraine Foundation. (2022b, November 29). *Migraine home Remedies | American Migraine Foundation.* https://americanmigrainefoundation.org/resource-library/migraine-home-remedies/

Booth, S. (2023, February 13). *Migraines vs. Chronic Migraines.* WebMD. https://www.webmd.com/migraines-headaches/chronic-migraines-explained#:~:text=Most%20people%20who%20are%20prone,a%20normal%20life%20a%20challenge.

Cluster headaches. (2024, February 22). Johns Hopkins Medicine. https://www.hopkinsmedicine.org/health/conditions-and-diseases/headache/cluster-headaches#:~:text=Cluster%20headaches%20are%20rare%20when,may%20last%20%20months%20or%20years.

Embr Labs. (n.d.). *Personal Temperature Control | EMBR Wave.* https://embrlabs.com/?utm_source=goog&utm_medium=paid&utm_campaign=e

mbr&gclid=CjwKCAjwy8i0BhAkEiwAdFaeGMPxut1rOqrKlMlTG0fcNLvCUK
HTruDhMXbuNZosiy3H4kBmUswTGRoC38kQAvD_BwE

Family and Medical Leave Act. (n.d.). DOL.
https://www.dol.gov/agencies/whd/fmla

McDermott, A. (2024, April 24). *15 natural ways to reduce migraine symptoms.*
Healthline. https://www.healthline.com/health/natural-ways-to-reduce-migraines

Medical devices - The Migraine Trust. (2022, May 13). The Migraine Trust.
https://migrainetrust.org/live-with-migraine/healthcare/treatments/medical-
devices/

Medication overuse headaches - Symptoms and causes - Mayo Clinic. (2023,
February 28). Mayo Clinic. https://www.mayoclinic.org/diseases-
conditions/medication-overuse-headache/symptoms-causes/syc-
20377083#:~:text=Medication%20overuse%20headaches%20%E2%80%94%20a
lso%20known,week%2C%20they%20may%20trigger%20headaches.

Mph, E. M. (2022, November 12). *Migraine symptoms by stage.* WebMD.
https://www.webmd.com/migraines-headaches/migraine-
phases#:~:text=Prodromal%20phase%20(before%20the%20migraine,Postdromal
%20phase%20(after%20the%20migraine)

*Preventive vs. abortive medication for chronic migraine: What you need to
know.* (2023, March 3). Health Central. Retrieved July 14, 2024, from
https://www.healthcentral.com/condition/migraines/preventive-vs-abortive-
medication-for-chronic-
migraine#:~:text=Medication%20Options%20for,Dr.%20Hindiyeh%20says.

WeatherX earplugs. (n.d.). https://www.weatherx.com/

Whitecoat. (2020, July 17). *Are there different types of migraine?* Regional
Neurological Associates. https://regionalneurological.com/different-types-of-
migraine/#:~:text=8%20Types%20of,see%20your%20neurologist.

Yaccarino, B. (2022, February 10). *Be Your Own Health Advocate: Why It's
Important & How to Do It Well.* United States of Healthcare.
https://unitedstatesofhealthcare.com/why-is-it-important-to-be-your-own-health-
advocate/